Prevent

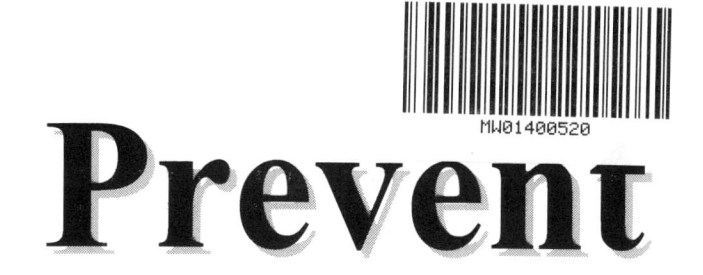

Cancer

With Mind & Spirit

Dr. Mark W. Tong

Spiritual Teacher & Healer

©2012 by Mark Tong, Inc.

All rights reserved.

Reproduction or translation of any part of this work beyond that permitted by Section 107 or 108 of the 1976 United States Copyright Act without permission of the copyright owner is unlawful. Requests for permission or further information should be address to: General Manager, Mark Tong, Inc.

This publication is designed to provide accurate and authoritative information in regarding the subject matter. It is sold with the understanding that the publisher is not engaged in rendering medical or psychological services or opinions. If medical or mental services or assistance is required, the services of qualified, competent professionals should be sought.

Any resources referenced in this work are done so only as a convenience to the reader and in no way consists an endorsement from the publisher. Publisher may directly or indirectly be compensated by any resource as an affiliate, common ownership, manager or contractor of such resource.

Printed in the United States of America

*For Dr. Carlos Garcia, MD, the entire staff and
patients at Utopia Wellness,
for allowing the opportunity to serve.
Blessings...*

How This Book Came About And Why Is It Really Important To Your Health

Dr. Mark W. Tong assists others in healing Spiritually. When he was offered the opportunity to help out an alternative cancer treatment center he quickly discovered something very startling …

Each patient experienced an emotional event or series of emotional events within thirty days of the first symptom and because of the patient's choice in viewing and responding to the event(s) it led to the manifestation of cancer.

"Dis-ease" is a result of being not-at-ease"

In each situation you have a choice: to be at ease or not. This book reveals the Spiritual ideas and views so that you can be "at ease" in every situation, promoting your wellness so that disease (dis-ease) cannot exist.

Enjoy!

Table of Contents

1	Introduction	7
2	What Causes Cancer	19
3	Healing Statements	23
4	Spiritual Ideas for Wellness	30
5	Questions for Patients & Clients	40
6	Conditions of Dis-ease	53
7	Seven Ideas for Wellness	73
8	First Symptom	103
9	Why Sharks Do Not Get Cancer	117
	Bonus Resources & Classes	122

CHAPTER ONE

Introduction

I was born with the knowing of how to assist people in healing and had a genuine understanding of the manifestation process and the Law of Attraction. What I found early in life was that the same process that one might use for health also works for wealth and peace of mind.

About 15 years ago, I started focusing and accelerating in the practice of assisting people in healing. It was just over a year ago that I was contacted through Facebook from a person that I had assisted in a healing over seven years ago, who asked if she could refer patients to me. And, I responded, "Sure, why not?"

Embarking on this new journey with these patients, I would see them in my office, or occasionally a home visit would be required. I worked spiritually with them being led by the Spirit myself. Several weeks went by and she contacted me again and asked if I would like to come in sometime to see where she worked, and if I would like to meet the doctor, Dr. Carlos Garcia, M.D., who runs an alternative cancer clinic, Utopia Wellness Center. I agreed.

My meeting with Dr. Garcia and his staff was brief, but I had time to explain who I was and what I did. To wrap-up this meeting, I pointedly asked him, "What can I do for you?" His response was, "Well, let me introduce you to some patients."

He took me back into his clinic and introduced me to a patient. I started immediately working on her, spiritually by understanding her beliefs and adding energy I worked on getting her to be "at ease". When I finished my session, he turned to me and said, "Look, here's the deal. You can come and go, and do anything you can do to help the patients."

So, I started working out of this alternative cancer treatment center. Normally, in my practice up until then, we would go right into working on the spiritual side of the healing. We would go right into such as adding energy, clearing it and moving forward with it. But this was more "mainstream" (even thought it was holistic and alternative), I had to evaluate each of the patient's beliefs and their belief system and incorporate those beliefs into bringing them "at ease" so that they would begin to heal.

"Heal the Mind First"

I quickly learned that with each and every one of these patients, I needed to go ahead and **heal the mind first** by bringing them at peace with themselves. Once the mind was healed and they had peace, then we could work on the Spirit and body using Divine energy, Love and Principle for healing.

Interestingly, after working with the patients for just a few weeks I was quite amazed with what I found.

First of all, I found that 100% of patients that I met with, we had been able to identify an event or series of events that occurred within 30 days of a physical condition's first appearance. That means within 30 days of the first symptom, they had an event or a series of events that was highly emotional, highly identifiable that it was linked to their physical condition.

Cancer is strictly a "mind issue."

Now, we're talking 100% of the patients! In addition, if they had an issue twenty years prior and they had some treatment then, for this condition, but then ten years later it appeared again, we were able to identify the emotional events that took place in both situations.

At first, because I'm psychic intuitive, I could use my intuitive abilities to go right to the root cause of their illness.

However, once doing this my concern was how could I duplicate myself? How could I show other people how to do this on their own? Not everyone has developed his or her intuitive abilities to the level needed for this type of work. So, I started incorporating kinesiology and muscle testing. Kinesiology is a method where you can access information from a patient that they may not be aware of consciously. The benefit was that not only would I be able do it, but almost anybody who wanted to could do it, and eventually even patients were learning how to muscle test themselves.

Special FREE Bonus Class

Learn kinesiology, muscle testing quick and easily with our free online video class at: http://www.BonusClass.com/

In the past, the process of identifying the issue or the series of events with a patient could take weeks.

Over the years I developed a formula or a process so we could identify most of our patient's issue(s) within one hour. By the end of that time, the patients would agree with our assessment. I'm saying the moment we brought it to their consciousness, to their awareness, and that we were to be in 100% agreement that the event(s) was tied to **their manifestation of their cancer, we were able to move forward.**

First, we would identify the emotional event(s) that caused them to be "not at ease," and once we were able to change their view of those situations or those events and change their emotions bonded to those event(s), **they began to heal.** The healing indicators would show up in blood tests, various medical tests, their level of energy and through muscle testing.

Also, in working with these patients, I noticed there were these identifiable patterns, these established patterns where each and every patient would fall into a group or a category. The "mind treatment" for that category was very similar (usually treated through guided meditations). At one particular time, I had an epiphany. It was my "aha" moment, right in the middle of assisting a patient. The idea came to me that if patients understood that these events caused their illness and they knew how to deal with it, they would never be sitting in front of me. I would never have seen them. They would be well and healthy. **They would be whole, pure, perfect, and disease-free.**

Another discovery working with these patients that was kind of startling, but needs to be brought to the forefront of your awareness. This discovery is that for most patients, there is a **benefit** to their disease, conscious or unconscious, though mostly unconscious of this. The patient doesn't realize that they hold this belief. An example of this is a person who does not like their occupation and can't face it, so he/she manifests a physical issue, and therefore doesn't have to go to work. Another example might be when spouse that doesn't listen to him/her doesn't give them any attention, isn't high on the spouses' "chart" or the "priority list," so all of this begins to manifest cancer in order to overcome this situation. The patient's hope is in manifesting a physical issue, they get that person's attention, they're heard, and they get higher on the priority chart.

The other amazing thing I discovered is that this transformation can be both real and unreal, occurred or not occurred. It could be just a thought. The body responds emotionally to something that is real or not. That is why if you wake up in the middle of the night with a cold sweat and your heart pounding because of a bad dream, the dream was not real. But the body responds as if it were. The same goes for a patient that believes their spouse no longer loves them or is cheating on them. I've worked with patients where I've asked, "Do you know it's real? Is it true? Do you know it's true?" It doesn't even have to be real and the body is responding. Just by meeting with these patients and speaking with them, as an intuitive, I can tell the moment when their body begins to constrict and not go into a "healing mode" that this is an "issue".

In this real/unreal situation, what happens is every time something reminds them of that event(s), and that emotion tied to the event(s), their body to responds to it, consciously or not. This means that every time the response is triggered by a thought, the patient goes into "un-healing," "dis-easing" and "not at ease" mode. In order to prevent this and to prevent dis-ease manifestation, what we need to do is be "at ease," and in this book, I will reveal the different groups of patients I encounter, and how to avoid being a patient yourself, the mindset, the culture, the spiritual beliefs that you may want to consider to incorporate into your life to promote wellness.

If you are at peace, dis-ease cannot exist.

The number one cause of cancer is your choice in **allowing something to take your peace away**, and that peace is taken either by anger, regret, remorse, resentment, fear, and un-forgiveness with yourself, or with others, past, present, future, real or not.

Now, the great thing is because our reality of the situation is subjective, to change our view of a situation or event(s), it does not have to be real, just believed or 'felt' which we do most often spiritually.

For example, if someone has negative financial issues, and they knew that these financial issues would be resolved shortly, real or not, (without them dying), they would be at peace. Our emotional and mental response then would determine our health and long-term ability to be at peace with any situation.

If someone has relationship issues and they believe that the situation can be or is resolved, just accepting this notion, or thinking they can change their situation they can arrive at place of peace.

The key to wellness for patients is for them to visualize themselves at peace at all costs, immediately, because once they do, they begin to heal. Visually, you can see the difference. Energetically, you can tell the difference. With muscle testing, you can tell the difference. With medical testing you can tell the difference.

What I'm about to reveal to you is the **mindset**, the **ideas**, and the **beliefs** that you can incorporate, so that you remain at peace. First, you do not allow yourself to let something or someone to take your peace away. Secondly, when you are confronted with a challenge, you choose peace instead of allowing something to take your peace, causing you to manifest dis-ease.

One thing I learned from Dr. Carlos Garcia is that cancer is a symptom. My belief from my observation is cancer is a symptom from **negative thinking** or "stinking thinking," (not having positive thoughts or a positive outlook) and if we can eliminate the "stinking thinking," disease will not exist.

This is quite a lot to mentally wrap your mind around, so I congratulate you for taking this step forward to being proactive, to being disease-free, and God bless.

Summary Chapter One
"Introduction"

- **Heal The Mind First**
- **Cancer is the result of emotional event(s)**
- **For healing, identify the events**
- **There is a benefit of the manifestation of cancer**
- **If you are at Peace – dis-ease cannot exist.**

This book reveals the mindset, the ideas and beliefs that YOU can incorporate to obtain Peace.

Bonus Class: Get your **FREE Bonus Class** at:
http://www.BonusClass.com

Chapter Two

What Causes Cancer?

"It's not what goes into your mouth that causes cancer. It's what comes out of your mouth. Or, what doesn't come out of your mouth and you hold and you bury and you stuff down into your consciousness."

Diet does play a role, but it's not the cause. The cause of cancer is **"stinking thinking."** I see patients who eat well, they exercise, might even be vegan or vegetarian, but they have a cancer issue.

When I first started working with patients, I quickly discovered that the commonality of all of the patients is **disharmony or discourse in their life.** There was something that they decided to allow to take their peace away. They chose to give up the peace of God for this thought. That's the common thread. 100% of all the patients that I've worked with had an emotional event or series of events that triggered the body into manifesting a physical issue. What I have seen is that triggering event is often within 30 days of the first symptom.

It might be a "loss of..." issue, such as a loss of a spouse, loss of a family member, loss of a house, loss of a job, loss of a 401k, loss of identity, real or unreal, imagined or not, but it is all too often tied to a loss. Additionally, the same response can occur due to a change, a change in household members, people coming, people going, change of corporate ownership, change of political office (Republican/Democrat), change of financial status (loss of income or wealth), or a changed view. They no longer view that child that way, their spouse that way, the government that way, their finances that way.

So, it's either a "loss of" issue or a type of change, a disruption of their life as they know it and a disruption of their sense of peace. Additionally, it might also be a loss of personal identity. They no longer see themselves as "that" person. Or, it might be the change in which they see another person, a family member, spouse, co-worker, or themselves.

The Role of Fear

So, what happens if there is an event or a series of events that invokes fear (fear is just one of the emotions that challenges one's peace), this fear might invoke a **false belief.** Mother passed away from this, Grandmother passed away from that. All of a sudden, you're celebrating an anniversary or you turn a certain age. Regardless, something triggers the idea and next thing you know is the person has manifested dis-ease.

The brilliant thing about all of this is it's all based on a chosen view, how you decide, how you choose to view a situation, your perception! When you change your perception to the positive (loving) you begin to heal. So, in 100% of the cancer patients that I've worked with, they all had an event or a series of events that they emotionally responded to, which manifested into dis-ease. Also, 100% of them, consciously or unconsciously had seen a benefit in having the dis-ease, and 100% of the patients are working with life lessons.

Chapter Two Summary
"What Causes Cancer"

- Diet plays a role but is not the cause.
- The common thread is discourse.
- Change your "view" of the event(s)
- The role of fear
- 100% of the patients …
- Dealing with an emotional event(s)
- Dealing with the your "choice" of view
- Saw a benefit to disease (unconsciously)
- Are dealing with a "life lesson"

CHAPTER THREE

Healing Statements

Now, I'd like to go over some statements, just so we're clear on some ideas, and the first two statements are ideas that I learned from working with Dr. Carlos Garcia in Oldsmar, Florida. The first one is that **cancer does not equal death.** Birth equals death. Your parents conceiving eventually equates to death. But, unfortunately society has solidified the connection that "cancer equals death." And, what happens when the patient hears that word, they associate it unfavorably. They also put themselves in a position of fear, and **fear fuels disease.**

If you ever want to increase the manifestation process in reverse, just add fear. **The first thing to overcome is the idea that cancer does not equal death.** Birth equals death. Because you were born, you will die. Because you have cancer doesn't mean you are going to die from cancer.

Secondly, another statement I learned from Dr. Garcia is that **cancer is just a symptom**. It's not the dis-ease. The dis-ease comes from the way you interpret events and the emotions you've tied to those events. It's your view of the event(s) and the emotions that you've tied to those events that your body is responding to.

The third idea is that **cells respond to emotions, not genetics.** We have this illusion that says that because our parents had it (disease, a condition, or something else) and our grandparents also had it, that we have a probability of getting it. That's not true. What goes from generation to generation to generation is **the idea**. The thought is what goes from generation to generation. The cells in your body do not know what your parents or grandparents had. It makes no difference to them.

What will make a difference to your cells are your emotions. Are you positive? Are you negative? Cancer is a symptom of **"stinking thinking."** Another concept we should focus on is that fact that **you are not a victim.** Since you choose the thoughts associated with event(s) you are a victim of your own thoughts. Since you brought it upon yourself, you cannot be a victim. It doesn't randomly select you. You select "it." It doesn't randomly fly through the air and say, "Hey, I'll take this person and that person and give them this 'issue' in this part of their body." It doesn't work that way. The way it works is you manifest it, consciously or unconsciously. Now, consciously, most people would say they would not manifest such an issue. Unconsciously however, you actually often do.

The other things I've found is that you unconsciously manifest it for a reason. Let me give you some actual reasons that I come across every day. First of all, if the person wants to be heard and nobody's listening to them, manifesting an issue like cancer seizes the attention they are seeking. A person who thinks that other family members are not listening them might think that by having cancer people begin listening to them. So, gaining attention is another thing that unconsciously manifests disease.

Remember when you were a small child and you had an issue and you stayed home from school and you got special treatment. What did you learn? You learned that physical conditions are tied to special treatment. Another important thing to bring to awareness is that physical conditions get you out of "stuff." What happened when you were a child? You didn't have to go to school. What if we have somebody who doesn't like his or her workplace? You're going to read about this a little later, if you don't like your workplace or your view of your workplace has changed, and you manifested a physical issue, you no longer have to go to that workplace. You are excused, a socially acceptable excuse, no questions asked.

So, there is a benefit from it, consciously or unconsciously. If you feel that you're in a situation, a life situation and there's no way out, whether it's in a relationship, financial, by manifesting this issue, there's a way out. Now remember, it's occurring consciously and unconsciously. Consciously, you probably wouldn't want to manifest it. Unconsciously, your reasoning is it is a way out. So, you're not a victim. It's chosen. It's manifested, and there are perceived benefits.

Another observation I have made is that people who are often dealing with physical issues are also dealing with and overwhelmed with a separate life issue. **It's a life lesson.** I can guarantee you this. 100% of the patients that I've met with and I've worked with were dealing with a life lesson. I promise you, it is a life lesson. I can also promise you that in my experience with patients I have identified what the "lesson" is. I have also identified how to shift a person's point of view so they can deal with that lesson more effectively.

All of the patients that I have worked with feel that due to the dis-ease they have encountered, they are closer to God. They are closer to the Universal source; they're closer to *their* source. There are "no atheists in foxholes," as the saying goes. Well, there are no atheists in cancer clinics either. They become closer to God. It's a benefit. And, later on, I am going to show you how to knock that benefit out so it doesn't even come in, consciously or unconsciously, into your thought process.

Then, the final statement I want to go over with you is that in 100% of the patients I've worked with, we have identified an event or series of events that occurred, and it is an emotional event, that occurred within 30 days of the first symptom. Now, I know patients are told by the medical community, "Oh, you had it in your body for years." Yes, you might have had it in your body for decades. Yes, you had it in your body all your life, since you were three years old, and we can test you and find that out to be true.

But, here's the "aha" moment - There is an emotionally significant event(s), what I like to call the tipping point, and it might not necessarily be the biggest point, but it's the point that takes you over the edge, where the event literally manifests into a physical issue. I cannot emphasize this anymore than I have! In my experience this occurs 100% of the time. Within 30 days of physical symptom, there was an event or a series of events that created an emotion, which manifested into the condition.

Chapter Three Summary
"Healing Statement"

- Cancer does not equal death
- Cancer is a symptom
- Cells respond to emotions
- You are not a victim
- Understand there are benefits
- It is a "life lesson"
- Cancer makes you closer to God

References:

"Cancer is a Symptom: The Real Cause Revealed (Volume 1)" **by Carlos M. Garcia, M.D.**

"The Biology of Belief: Unleashing the Power of Consciousness, Matter, & Miracles" **by Bruce H. Lipton**

CHAPTER FOUR

Spiritual Ideas for Wellness

Here are some spiritual ideas for wellness. If it resonates with you or matches your beliefs, that's great and if it does not, that's okay too. It is what I found that people who have particular mindsets are more conducive to healing. I also noticed in dealing with patients and clients that have these ideas incorporated in their belief system enjoy a much rapid healing process.

Let's go over some ideas. Again, if it resonates with you, great if it does not, that's okay. The first view is your view of God. I found that people who believe that God is punishing, would punish themselves. Those who believe that God is love or unconditional love heal much faster. There's less fear. **That Divine Love casts out fear**. And remember, fear is one of the chief components, contributors to dis-ease.

When a doctor tells you, you have this or that, and it is going to progress this way, all this fear is brought into play immediately. It actually results in the opposite of healing. To cast out fear, we use Divine Love. So, if your view of God is unconditional love, it's a real easy step for you.

For Christians, I also look to see what their view of Jesus is. Now, if their view of Jesus is that Jesus is the Son of God, I turn to them and ask them, "Well, then who are you?" And, they say, "Well, I'm also a child of God." Now for these people, it's easier to heal because there is no identity issue once they realize who they really are and who the Creator really is: that they are a spiritual being in a body, and that that **spiritual being that's in the body has dominion over the body**. Once they realize they have dominion over the body, what can't they heal?

The other challenge for us is found on page two of Genesis that states, "And behold, everything that was created was very good." Well, the challenge is that if we see everything that was created as "very good," you're more conducive to wellness and to healing. Now, if you believe in darkness, in the power of darkness, or the "fallen angel" and all that, then here is another idea to contemplate: If you give God's power to darkness, it's more of a challenge for healing. Let me explain.

Here is the way I look at darkness and I try to see if the patient or client will agree with the idea that there's only one "Source" or Higher Power. For me, there's only one power and that's God. Now, if they believe God is good or God is love, then where does darkness come from?

In response, I usually hear about the story of the falling angel. Well, here's my theory, whether it's true or not, whether you believe it or not, whether you want to buy into it or not, I don't really care. Is my position conducive to wellness? Yes. I believe any dark power is an entity that has tricked us to taking God's power and giving it away to them, and it's not our job to give God's power to anything. If something doesn't have any power, it cannot harm you. If you do not give it any power, it cannot harm you.

But, we give power away all day. We give it to our politicians. We give it to people. We give it to doctors. We give it to dis-ease. If you take the power away and give it back to God, believing that there's only one power, you're on the way to healing. If a particular person is what you've chosen to take your peace away, then you can take the power away from that person and give it back to God. I also find it with spouses, where there's an abusive relationship or something that is still haunting the client or patient. We take the power away. Energetically through meditation we can literally take the perceived power away the person or organization that might have influence over the patient, bringing the patient peace regarding the situation.

It is not your job to give God's power to anything.

We often talk about darkness, evil and the dark side. My belief for wellness is if you can see there's only one Creator, you can see there's only one power, and then everything that was created is very good and still is very good. If you can agree that it is not our job to give God's power away to any entity, then you're on the way to wellness.

Is this heaven or is it hell?

I ask each and every one of my clients and patients: "Is this physical plane that we're occupying, is it heaven or is it hell or a little bit of both?" No matter how they answer, they're right. But, how they answer also shows me their mindset, and if they see it as hell, then they are suffering. In heaven, it's healing. It's wellness. It's wholeness. So, when a person sees this physical plane as "in heaven," dis-ease cannot exist and it is a choice of how you wish to view it.

For Christians, most of them are at church every Sunday mumbling through The Lord's Prayer. They recite a portion of that famous prayer, "on Earth as it is in heaven." My belief is that when Jesus talked about the kingdom, He didn't mean that He had to die to get there. You don't have to die to get to a heavenly state. Heaven is right here. And, everybody says, "Oh, this isn't heaven." Well, it's like heaven. How about that? Would you buy that? Because, if you believe that it's like heaven, dis-ease cannot exist, and it's your choice how to view it.

Then, sometimes I get a patient or client that looks for the exception. A patient every now and then asks me, "What about the two year-old that gets killed?" Well, I have a response to that. I don't care if you believe in it or not, but it's healing and it explains a lot, and that is we are all here on this physical plane to learn lessons. And, yes, it's tragic that the two year-old child may get shot in a drive-by shooting. But, it's in order, and here's the theory...

There's a theory that I use and it is what is called Sacred Contracts. Prior to your arrival on this physical plane, you and God get together and you say, "Look, I'm going to go down to Earth and there are things I need to learn." God then picks your parents, spouse(s), your lifestyle, your status; God picks everything for your lesson(s). Then you sign off on the whole deal. They are all there for a lesson. And so, when the two year-old gets shot, and we say it's tragic, (because it is tragic), we can also see that it's in Divine Order. All the people involved agreed to it accepting such circumstances, and they agreed to it for a life lesson and the child gave its life for others to learn this lesson.

Every single patient and client that I meet that has a major challenge with their health, are dealing with a **life lesson**. And, it's real easy in dealing with patients with challenging health situations, is to look back and say, "Well, what is the life lesson?" As we look back we often see that it is repeating, and it repeats until they learn it.

When we ask ourselves, "What is that life lesson?" And once we understand it and we turn it around, it cancels it out. When we change our view of the situation, it cancels it out. If we are working with forgiveness, well then, forgive. Looking to surrender and that is what we're working on, then surrender, give it up. If it's trust in God, shift and have trust in God.

In dealing with the "heaven and hell thing," here are some tricks. One…First of all, if you go out in the middle of the night on a clear night and you look up at the stars, they're all in order. When you walk through nature, can you say, "Hey, this is heaven!" Well, when you're not in nature and you're in the big city, it's all in Divine Order. It is heaven. It is a choice, and **when you see it as heaven, dis-ease cannot exist.**

Another trick for wellness, (super powerful), is to see yourself one year from today. See yourself at peace. Really visualize you being at peace. Another trick to really turbo charge your wellness, is to project yourself, go sit somewhere in silence, project yourself one year from today and observe your family, friends, faith, finances, and your fitness. The reason why this is so powerful is that when your conscious is full of bliss or a blissful state in which you're manifesting, **dis-ease in the unconscious will not be present.**

Your unconscious has a direction now, because consciously, you have set peace in motion and action in that direction and everything in the Universe starts coming together so it will happen, and it won't even be a year from now. It happens immediately. Things start coming about in your favor.

My theory for wellness is when you see yourself in the future at peace, your body instantly heads towards that direction, and when it's in that direction, dis-ease does not exist. Your unconscious doesn't have a clean slate to make up its own mind to take you in a different direction.

So, the ideas and the concepts for wellness is first of all, your view of God. If God is love, unconditional love, that's healing. It casts out fear. If you are Christian, your view of Jesus is that He's the Son of God, and you too are a son or daughter of God. Identity issues will never come into your life. An identity issue is a major reason for disease. The housewife with the empty nest who doesn't know what she is now, or a corporate executive who gets forced into retirement or the company is downsized and he/she doesn't have that identity anymore, are examples of identity issues.

Chapter 4 Summary
"Spiritual Ideas For Wellness"

- **View of God**
- **View of Jesus**
- **Everything created is "very good"**
- **Don't give God's Power away**
- **Heaven or Hell?**
- **Life Lessons**
- **See Peace 1 year from today.**

CHAPTER FIVE

Questions For Patients & Clients

Each time I meet with a new patient or client, there's a series of questions I usually use to begin interviewing them to see where they are in their beliefs. I need to understand their beliefs because **all beliefs become real.** The first questions I usually have for a patient or a client are, "What is your spiritual and religious experience? What is your background?"

The reason why I ask these questions is because I need to know their starting point. The other reason why is I need to understand what beliefs they have, and how they view the world, so later on when I assist them in healing, I know which tools I can use or cannot use or cannot access. So, I ask them, again, "What's your spiritual and/or religious background?" I take notes on every question I ask. I keep very detailed notes, because I can refer back to them later on when we start assisting them in healing.

Then, the next question I ask is, "What's your view of God?" The reason I ask this is that a person's view of God is also their view of themselves. It will also give me insights on the expectations that are required for healing. As mentioned earlier, if somebody thinks that God is a punishing God, then often, they might be punishing themselves. If God is a loving God to this person, it makes it very easy for healing, because if God is loving, then God is forgiving. If God is forgiving, **God doesn't have a problem with you.** And, it breaks it down even more to where **only you have a problem with you.**

A person who views God as punishing is a lot more challenging in healing and it limits you on the spiritual tools that you can use later on. And, it's okay if that's their belief, but again, it limits the tools you can use in healing them spiritually. If they're Christian, then I add another question to the interview, and that's, "What's your view of Jesus? Who is he?" Now, often we get the answer, "He's our Lord and Savior." which is an okay answer, but it does limit some of the tools you might use later on in healing identity. So I re-word the question to be more specific. Is he God? Is he the Son of God? Who are you?

The one who says, "He's the son of God," then I ask, "Well, who are you?" And, here again, we are trying to see how people view themselves. A powerful tool later on to use is, if a Christian sees Jesus as the Son of God, I turn around and ask, "Well, who are you?" And, they think for a moment and then respond; "I'm also a son/daughter/child of God." Now that gives us a lot of spiritual tools for healing! "The Son of God does not have any dis-ease, so why do you?"

Once this is sorted out, identity is not an issue. The ability to receive is not an issue, and the real challenge in healing is whether they feel worthy to receive any healing? Do they feel worthy to be healed and to have wellness? This is a challenge. So, I do ask, "What are your spiritual and religious beliefs?" I ask them, "What's your view of God?" If they're Christian, I say, "Well then, what's your view of Jesus?" Then I go further and ask, "What is your view of yourself?" And, I try to sort it all out.

Then, my next big question is, "Time-wise, chronological order, exactly when did the first symptom appear? The first time that you got an idea that there might be a problem? When was that?" This time frame needs to be zeroed in on to a precise month and year. If a client doesn't recall exactly, the other question I ask each and every one of my clients and patients is, "Do I have their permission to muscle test them on their behalf?"

Muscle testing is kinesiology, where I can instantly, on their behalf, find out which month, what day of the month, if I need to know, did the first symptom appear, and I can run through their entire life and see when the first idea of this physical condition first appeared and when did it manifest into something.

My next question to the client or patient is, "What exactly was going on in your life at that time?" And, what I'm looking for is **chaos**. I'm looking for anything that's not at ease, something that they chose and allowed to take their peace away, and here's what I'm looking for. I'm listening for any betrayal issues, somebody moving, either somebody moving in or somebody moving out, a shift in culture, a change, or a life-changing event. I'm just looking for a key emotional trigger.

Now, here's the thing. It might not be the biggest event. They might have had, (and this is often), significant emotional event a few years ago, and it's been stuffed in their body and stuffed away unconsciously. Then, years later, something triggers the idea back to that time and place when that emotional event occurred. Their body automatically goes back to that same reaction and they manifest the physical issue.

So, it doesn't necessarily have to be the biggest emotional event, but it's what I call the tipping point. It's "the straw that breaks the camel's back". It's the final thing that makes the body say, "Hey, you need to wake up. You need to respond. You need to address this issue. You need to change your view of this issue." It is at that point where you decided to manifest it into a physical issue.

Now, I want to tell you that 100% of the clients and patients that I've met that had a physical issue had an emotional event just prior to the symptom. Now, the medical community says, "Yeah, you had this issue for years and this and this, but the question is: why did it just now manifest? Why did it just become an issue?

One day, I was speaking in front of a group of patients with cancer, and another family member who was accompanying the patient said that she had an "issue" about ten years ago, a physical issue, and she cannot believe she would choose to have disease. She couldn't believe that she brought it on herself, and she said this in front of the whole group, and she was at the far end of the room. I was at the other end of the room. I looked straight across at her, and when she told me what issues she had, I said, "What was going on with your family at that time?" You could just see that I hit a nerve with this person. It struck her heart from across the

45

room, and she looked right at me, and she said, "Yeah, but everybody has family issues. How come everybody doesn't get this physical issue?" I said, "Because not everybody chooses to view the situation and to respond to that emotional event the way you did, and you might have had a series of prior events that you'd just been stuffing, burying, not addressing, and finally, when we hit this tipping point, this incident occurred that took you over the top and it manifested into the physical issue."

So, among the series of questions that I ask is, "What exactly was going on in your life at that time when the first symptom appeared?" Now, whether they know consciously or unconsciously...Again, I use kinesiology, muscle testing on their behalf. In the beginning of doing this work, I was doing it from an intuitive level. I am an intuitive, so I can access other realms to find out the same information.

The challenge is, not everybody has built their intuitiveness to the level to where they can actually assist others. So, I can teach somebody to use muscle testing, and within seconds or minutes, we can identify the issue, who was the issue, who was involved with the issue and exactly when it happened. Another thing I want to point out is that when I do identify the issue, 100% of the patients and clients, when it's brought to their awareness, agree with me.

Now, at first, they might be in denial. At first, they say, "Well, there's no way I would manifest something because of this little old incident, or this emotional event." When we start working on it, we begin discussing it, we establish it to their conscious awareness. Again 100% of the patients and clients that I've worked with, when it's identified, agreed that this emotional event was the issue.

Another question I mentioned earlier (but is worth repeating) is to ask patients and clients, "Is this heaven or is it hell, or a little of both?" The reason why is the way they answer that question shows me their view of the world, and with a lot of my Christian clients and patients, they'll say, "No, this can't be heaven. Heaven is greater than this physical plane."

Then, I remind them that every Sunday, they mumble through The Lord's Prayer. The remainder of the conversation follows something like this:
Me: "Do you go to church?"
Client/Patient: "Yes."
Me: "Do pray The Lord's Prayer?"
Client/Patient: "Yes."
Me: "Well, in The Lord's Prayer, doesn't is say 'on Earth that it is in heaven'? Was Jesus trying to tell us that we don't have to die to enter the kingdom, and that the kingdom is here if we wish? Can we look at this physical plane as heaven or hell or a little bit of both, and everyone is right?"

Here's the "aha" for wellness, when you view this physical plane as heaven, dis-ease cannot exist. There is no dis-ease in heaven, and when you see this physical plane as heaven, dis-ease does not exist.

If you want the ultimate prayer for another person in healing, first of all, you need to see this world as heaven, and then you ask for that person, that friend that you're praying for to see the world a "little bit different," as in heaven.

When people make the "shift" and they begin to see this world as heaven, they see all the beauty surrounding us with gratitude. They become at peace, and with that peace, we find our healing beginning. **Dis-ease is you choosing to allow something to take the peace of God away from you.** When you go back and you see this world as heaven, again, dis-ease cannot exist.

Then, there are always those people who come to me "armed and ready" with the Bible. I always remind them that if they just read page 2 of Genesis, "And behold, it was very good," they understand that God is good and God is loving. They further understand and agree that everything God created is very good. If they truly understand these ideas, then they are on the road to wellness.

A short road to wellness is there's one Creator and everything that was created is very good. That Creator is loving, therefore the Creator is forgiving. The Creator doesn't play favorites. Everything that happens, happens for the better, even if we cannot see it from our perspective right away. There's one plan and it is God's plan, and that's a great plan. When you get hold of this notion and begin to understand it, the body shifts into being at peace and being well.

There is no negative part of life if you view this as heaven. A lot of times, I have to break it down to patients and clients. You walk through nature and everything is in divine order. Go out and look at the stars in the middle of the night on a clear night and see that it's all in divine order. Well, it's no different in the city. In nature you might see an anthill with all the ants coming and going as "in order". But, it might be much harder to see it in the city with everyone coming and going out of a large office building. It's no different wherever you are. It's all in order. It's all according to plan. And, if you see this physical plane as heaven, again, dis-ease cannot exist. There is no negativity.

Then, the final interview question, and it might be towards the end right before I work on treatment with a client or a patient, but that is, "Why are you here? Why are you on this physical plane? And, whatever it is, why aren't you doing it? From this point forward, you can be working with a clean slate. You can have a completely empty board. So, you can design your life."

It's back to the other question that I ask each and every patient, is, "Where are you going to be one year from now, doing what, and are you at peace?" And, if they don't see themselves a year from now, well, they might not be here a year from now, and if they don't see themselves at peace, they're not in the direction of healing. And, if they don't see that at this moment, nothing is more important than their health, they have a clean slate, so now is the time to design your new life where you are at peace.

Therefore, for wellness, you need to look forward to tomorrow, to next month, to next year, and you need to see yourself in a constant state of peace, and if you are, dis-ease cannot exist.

Chapter 5 Summary
"Questions for Patients & Clients"

- **Spiritual & Religious Background?**
- **View of God**
- **View of Jesus**
- **Who is Jesus?**
- **Who are you?**
- **Chronologically / First Symptom?**
- **Permission to Muscle Test?**
- **What chaos was going on then?**
- **Heaven / Hell / Both?**
- **Why are you here?**
- **Design your new life 1 year from now**

CHAPTER SIX

Conditions of Dis-ease

Another big factor to wellness or conditions in which people manifest dis-ease, is their personal finances. Over the last few years, the economy has been tough on almost everybody. People got hit hard. They lost their 401K's. They lost percentages of their retirement. They might have lost this, lost that, lost their home, or whatever. Their family members may also be in a tight situation. They're trying to help family members, put themselves in a better position, and they're running out of cash.

What happens is, maybe consciously or unconsciously, at some point of life, they decided that when they retire, they would have X amount of money, and when the money runs out, their goal is to die broke. I hear people say this all the time - the ultimate financial plan is when you spend your last dollar is on the last day you're here on this physical earthly plane.

Well, that's fine and dandy, but the challenge with that is, people have unexpectedly experienced a drop in finances, and when they get that drop, it naturally makes them not at ease with their situation and becomes a concern. Remember, if they don't have enough money, they won't have any food, shelter, and clothing. So, they might as well be dead. And so, the financial condition of a person actually plays a huge part on wellness.

Some ideas...First of all, if finances come up on the chart, you need to do everything you can to balance the budget. What other income can you pursue? What other assets can you access? What can you do? You must come up with a plan very quickly and implement it. Now, the challenge is your ego is going to say, "No." It falls under lost identity. If you lose your business because of the economy or you're no longer that person, if you lose your house, your boat, your car, whatever, that's your identity. You've attached your identity to all this "stuff." It is often that we see that people become **possessed with their possessions.**

We see it with business when they attach the business name to the person and they become that identity, and when that business is no longer around, they don't know who they are. So, they become the person with the **physical condition**. To counter this is to see that the Universe has always provided for you. I usually ask patients and clients, "God always provided for you. Everything you've asked for, you've gotten. So that's not going to change."

Second of all is, when you know who you really are, you know you're not that stuff. Remember the word "possession" means being "possessed", being possessed by objects, and so you need to work on knowing who you really are, the power and the abundance that you're really connected to, and you need to come up with an action plan immediately. If a person has a physical issue and it's the result of personal finances, they need to resolve it right now before healing takes place because it's still a problem. It's still in their mind.

It needs to be implemented immediately. If it means selling something, sell it. If it means moving somewhere, move there. If it means downsizing, downsize. The one thing about wellness is if health is high on your priority chart, then you need to make it a priority and nothing comes in front of it.

The next cause for dis-ease, are for all those people that are **carrying the world on their shoulders**. For some reason they take it upon themselves for being concerned about carrying the burdens of the world. It's not your world to carry. Universal law of possession says everything belongs to God. It belongs to God, and you don't have to carry it. The challenge with these patients or clients, with this part of the process, is that the people carrying the world think they're in control.

Patients and clients think they're in control, and they typically watch the news and they believe in the illusion that the world's coming to an end, and that they didn't do their job carrying the world. They're concerned about our children's future, and they take on so much of this responsibility of the world that they literally manifest dis-ease. To fix this, it's really easy. **It's not your world to carry. Turn it over to God.**

The next condition of dis-ease is the lost identification. The lost identification can be the empty nest syndrome for a housewife. She was a housewife, raised the children, now the children are now leaving the nest, going to college, and moving on. Who is she now? What is her identity? Or there's the corporate executive whose company gets downsized, so he/she gets forced into retirement, and goes out of business. Who is he now? Or you might lose stuff. Like your house or home, your business, your boat, your car, or whatever it is, and you just become this person of loss.

What happens is that unconsciously or consciously, you don't know who you are and you give your unconscious a clean slate to create whatever your unconscious thinks you should be, you might end up being the person with the physical issue. This is not conducive to wellness.

Here are some ideas for wellness in dealing with your identity. First of all, you're a **spiritual being**. Your soul was created by God at the beginning of time and will continue to be here to eternity. Your soul was created by God. For the Bible readers, Genesis, "And, on the seventh day, God rested." Everything was done. It was complete, nothing more to do. So, that means your soul and that soul essence has been here since the beginning and will continue to be around forever. That's who you really are. That's your true inheritance.

I mentioned earlier that Christians and their view of Jesus who is the Son of God, have the belief that "Even the least among us can do all that I can do and even greater things." So, you begin to internalize that. You're no longer that person with the "stuff." You're no longer the person with the "dis-ease." If you knew who you really were, and if you knew what you were really connected to, and if you really knew who walked beside you, dis-ease could not exist.

The next group for wellness is **false belief.** False belief is akin to the person who sneezes while somebody on the other side of the room also starts to sneeze. They think the germs went across the room and infiltrated the body, and now they sneeze. No, it's like yawning. If a person on one side of the room yawns, then the person on the other side of the room yawns. It wasn't because the yawning molecules went across the room, infiltrated that person's body, and caused them to yawn. What went across the room was the **idea**, the thought.

We see this in genetics. We put so much faith in genetics. However, **genetics is an illusion**. The cells in your body do not care what your parents had, your mother had, your father had, or your grandparents had. They don't know, don't care, and it does not matter. The cells in your body are responding to your emotions. Whether it's positive or negative, they're just responding. Your body is responding to your emotions and acting on it.

The reason why we know false belief isn't true is the medical community has to speak in percentages. The reason why is, because it's **not** a science. **Modern medicine is not a science.** How many times do you hear a doctor say, "100%?" Never. The reason why is there's always these "outside" factors or external variables.

If the idea that illness is caused by genetics was so true, then why don't identical twins get the same illness? The reason why is that they interpret situations "differently." Let's say you have identical female twins. At age 17, they both go to the school dance. Now, they went to the same exact dance. One perceived it one-way. One perceived it another way.

One might have said, "I had a great time." The other one comes back and says, "I hate men." Throughout their life, they repeat the same thing where one had a great time and the other one hates men. They both get into a relationship and the one still hates men. The one that hates something manifests an issue and the one that enjoyed life doesn't get the issue. But, according to genetics, they both should have the issue. If one gets it, the other one does, but statistically, they don't. So, genetics is an illusion. It is all in how you choose to respond to situations.

When a doctor tells a patient they have X amount of days, months or years to live, that's a false belief, because there are cases where the doctor tells them they have three months to live, and they live ten years. You always hear the case where they tell the mother that she's going to die in three months, and she ends up living another fifteen years until her daughter gets married and then she dies. Or, the surgeon who does the procedure absolutely perfect, everything is perfect, and ten minutes later, the person passes on. We have all heard about the person who's in the car wreck, supposed to be dead, and still here.

Here is the deal. Your soul has dominion over the body. God gave your soul dominion over the body. The body has no dominion over you unless you give it to "it." So, we have all these things called false beliefs, "If this, then that." It is the reason why I mentioned you don't use medical terms. Don't run out and research everything on the Internet right away, because if it's nothing, it's nothing. If you give it no thought, it doesn't become anything.

I had a case where a lady came to me and said, "Hey, I'm really worried about my husband. He thinks he's going to pass on." Now, I've met her husband before and he wasn't that old, and I'm saying, "Well, what's going on?" She goes, "Well, he's ready to turn 50, and his father passed away when he turned 50, and his grandfather passed away when his grandfather turned 50, and he's getting ready to turn 50, so he thinks he's going to pass on.

The cells in your body do not know when your parents passed. What goes from generation to generation to generation is ideas. We see this with women labeled with breast cancer. Mom had it, so daughter's going to have it. If they have this one particular gene, they think they have a higher percentage of having it, and it's absolute.

If you didn't know this, you would not have that thought, consciously or unconsciously. If you think your mom had it, and so you're going to have it, the chances of you having it are increased because **all beliefs become real**. If you believe that there's a gene that's going to make you have an issue, that's not good, because you fell into the idea of false belief.

Here is the Spiritual approach to genetics. Who is your true parent? Not your biological parent, but who is your true parent? The one who created your soul? It's God. Well, God does not have an issue, any physical issue. That's your true inheritance. So, genetically, when you look at your true parent who is whole, pure and perfect, disease-free, that's who you really are, not your biological parents, your true parent.

The next type of challenge for awareness or type of patient, and it's one that I call **suicide**. If you think about it, people can't die of old age anymore. You've got to label something, and what better way to go than to manifest cancer.

If somebody wants to go, they cannot go down to the local bridge and jump off, or a high building and jump off the building, because if they did, they'd be considered coward, or they're told through religious or spiritual experience that committing suicide was a "no-no" because you won't go to heaven and this and that and all the other stuff (which suicide is not "cool"). However, on the other hand, it is socially acceptable for you to become a victim of a mainstream illness that you can pass from and nobody will question it. People will actually pity you. You will actually get special attention.

There are many different ways or different reasons why people manifest the suicidal condition of cancer, and the reason why is, first of all, they might want to **prove a point**. Believe it or not, patients want to prove a point. They're like Jesus on the cross. They give their life for mankind. Sometimes it is, their perception, it **is the only way out.** They are either in a relationship they can't get out of, and in their mind, they're in a box. So, they can't get out of the box. The only way out is to die, so they manifest it.

They may want revenge, get back or **punish somebody else,** it is perceived as a great way to do it. I see it all the time. You want to get back at a parent, a loved one, or yourself (guilt). They manifest an issue. They just get tired and they don't know anything else to do. They manifest an issue.

To overcome this idea is that when you're at peace with everybody around you, you're at peace with the people at work, you're at peace with your family members, you're at peace with yourself, and your connection to God is great, you won't be thinking this. It's not in your thought.

Another condition is our possession of **guilt of the past.** We see this with finances or because of their actions, people lost all of their money and they lost the family's money, or they led other people to lose money, and they feel guilty. So they come up with the idea to punish themselves and they manifest a disease.

I see it with females with abortion issues. I see it with people with past abuses, substance abuse, emotional abuse, and past actions and failures. The way to fix this is to ask them whether they think "God has a problem with you?" If God is all loving then God is all forgiving, so God does not have a problem with you. **You have a problem with you.** Self-forgiveness is a real big issue with wellness. If you did what you felt was right at that time. End it.

I heard the example of where you bring in this little child, and you ask the little child to do algebra, and he just looks at back at you and says, "Ah, I don't know what algebra is." You wouldn't hold it against him, because he just didn't know. But, you would hold things against yourself even though you did not know the issue at that time!

For wellness, if in every situation you are comfortable with your actions, you are comfortable with what you do and you're at peace with your actions, dis-ease won't exist. If you can see that God does not have a problem with you and you can forgive yourself of any past actions, then you are there.

I go through this series of questions with my clients. I usually ask, "Does God have a problem with you?" Now, if they say yes, then I go back to one of my questions, "What's your view of God?" If they say, "God is all loving and forgiving." Then God does not have a problem with you. And, if God does not have a problem with you, then you have a problem with you.

If somebody else has a problem with you, that's their problem. If God does not have a problem with you, then why do you have a problem with you? For most people, you're your toughest critic. Ask yourself this question, "Does God have a problem with my actions? Why do I have a problem with these actions?" And forgive yourself. Move on. It's not worth your health.

The next thing that takes people's peace away and manifests into disease is **betrayal** in relationships, real or unreal. The thing about betrayal is either it's the person who's betraying or the person who gets betrayed. Either one can lose the peace. The person who betrayed can **self-punish**. The person who was betrayed upon has **forgiveness** to deal with.

The biggest challenge with forgiveness is people associate forgiveness with "letting people go," not holding people accountable, and it's not. Forgiveness is when you don't hold it. You don't carry it. It's their problem. Forgiveness is a huge lesson on this physical plane, and often I remind Christian patients and clients of Jesus' last words, as he was on the cross, "Forgive them, Father, for they do not know…" And that is your self-forgiveness, "Forgive me, Father, for I did not know." If it's another person, it's "Forgive them, Father, for they did not know."

It doesn't mean you don't hold them accountable, but you don't hate them. The thing about betrayal is whether it's real or unreal, it is a **huge segment in dis-ease**. In the perception, the perception between the two individuals regarding betrayal, she says he cheated. You interview him and what he did in his mind was not cheating. It is similar to someone saying, "I did not have sexual relations..." Well, he did or did not have sexual relations depending on definitions.

I get this with the females, thinking they had relationships. They tell me about all their relationships, and often, their relationships are one-night relationships. If I were to interview the male, his perspective would be, "No, it wasn't a relationship." He just got lucky.

So, there's this discourse on what is cheating, what is not cheating, these gaps in perception, and the thing is, whether it's real or unreal, your body is responding.

In any situation you have only three options. You can **accept** that's what it was or **"what is."** You can try to **change** the situation or change the person in the situation, or **avoid it**. But, it is a huge component to the physical issue of cancer.

Another huge segment of patients and clients is what I call the **"messed up family"**. The messed up family is usually ego-based. You're dealing with a life lesson. The reason why I say it is ego-based is because you, as a parent, or you, as a family member, should've, would've, could've done something different so the family or a family member would not be "so messed up" or they're a reflection of your parenting. They're a reflection of your family. They disgraced the family, they disgraced the family name, and being "not at peace" within the family is huge. It is a big leading factor for dis-ease.

When I muscle test someone, one of the first questions is, "Is it in the family or out of the family?" The chances of it being within the family are huge, because we're talking emotions. We're also talking about things over a long period of time, and just repeating and repeating. The messed up family is a reflection of your identity, or you've allowed it to be a reflection of your identity, and to let it go is to acknowledge the Universal Law of possession, and the Universal Law of possession says all the family members belong to God. Now, if you have children, you have responsibilities, but you also can turn them over to God too, because they belong to God. You are just entrusted with them for a short period of time.

Also, when there is a shift in the household, either somebody coming or somebody going, it can play a role on somebody's peace. It plays a role energetically.

To fix the messed up family perspective is the realization that first of all, you did what you did. You did the best you could do. It's the best you could do under that situation. Or, it's their problem. I no longer have to carry the world. Whatever it is, you only have three options. You can either **accept it**, which "that's the way it is," **change** whatever you can, or **avoid** it at all costs.

Chapter 6 Summary
"Conditions of Dis-ease"

- **Loss of finances**
- **Carrying the world**
- **Identity**
- **False Belief**
- **Suicide**
- **Prove a point**
- **Punish**
- **Guilt**
- **Betrayal**
- **Messed Up Family**
- **Attention / Control**

CHAPTER SEVEN

Seven Ideas for Wellness

I'd like to go over some ideas for preventing any disease and accepting wellness. The first idea on the chart is literally life changing. It's something I can guarantee you or I can promise you that if you incorporate it in your life, it truly does promote wellness. This necessity is **meditation.**

When you set your alarm clock 15 or 20 minutes earlier than normal, and you get up early, and you go sit in a space that you set aside for meditation, whether it's on a pillow on the floor or in a chair, maybe you'd light a candle, but it's a designated spot for you to connect with the Divine, the Source, God. And, the reason why meditation is so powerful is it solves and it fixes a lot of issues regarding wellness or dis-ease.

First of all, when you sit there in silence and you connect with the source, you begin to experience the peace of God, and with the peace of God, this is one thing I can promise you, **dis-ease**

cannot exist, because the opposite of peace is not being at-ease and that is what your cells in your body respond negatively to, is that "not at ease." When you begin each morning by being at ease, you're reminded throughout the day to be at ease, and the more at ease you become, the more it promotes wellness.

So, I suggest that you set the clock 15, 20 minutes early, designate a spot for meditation. Either sit on the floor with a pillow or in a chair, but comfortably, and get quiet with yourself and connect with the source.

Another reason why meditation is so powerful is that many people who are dealing with a dis-ease, are dealing with identity issues, whether it's the housewife who is now an empty-nester, the corporate executive who just got downsized or forced into retirement, in either case, they no longer know who they are, and when they no longer know who they are, they become not at ease. When someone becomes not at ease, it allows the unconscious mind to create a new identity, and they become the person with the issue.

So, my theory is, when you know who you truly are, and are truly connected to that source, dis-ease cannot exist. Identity is not an issue, because you know who you are. Also meditation, a form of prayer, my belief in prayer is that God's job is done and God is all-knowing, so in prayer there is nothing tell God to do, you just listen.

So, what we're doing in prayer is, we're asking ourselves to see a situation differently. We're asking to see the world through God's eyes. It's "God, let me see this differently." Because my theory is based on the way God sees the world - **it's all in order**. There is no chaos. It's all in order, according to God's plan. If you see everything all in order, dis-ease cannot exist. So, in meditation, often, if something is bothering us, something we're concerned with, we're just asking to view it differently. "Allow me to see it through God's eyes."

The real key thing to meditation is it makes you closer to God. One of the benefits to dis-ease is that it makes the patient closer to the source. It makes them closer to God. The idea is if you meditate and you begin to get closer to God, there is no reason for dis-ease to exist. That benefit has been removed. The identity benefit has been removed. So, for wellness, the top of the chart is to meditate. As Jesus said, "Sit in the closet alone in silence."

I had somebody once tell me they didn't like sitting alone in silence, and my response was quite simple. "Because, when you sit there alone in silence, you don't like the person you are with." Meditation makes you, or forces you to be comfortable with who you really are. In that silence you can also reflect. So, again, I put meditation as number one action you can take.

For prevention – the number two idea is a very simple one. I do prescribe this to every single patient I have received. It's something I know to be true, and that is to **turn off the news**. Disconnect yourself from the news media. First of all, the media is not true. It's not real. Second of all, it's not positive.

Your body responds to positive thoughts and emotions. If you watch the news, your body is not responding in a positive way. It is not healthy. It is the media's opinion of reality. It is not a reflection of how God sees the world. Remember that the news has to invoke fear. If they invoke fear, they have your attention and they have control over you. **Fear is a source of dis-ease.** It's the biggest fuel. So, what is the purpose of watching the news, or listening to the media the media?

Let me tell you the way it works. If something were to happen, somebody will tell you and they can't wait to tell you. I had a person come up to me and say, "Well, how do you know what's going on?" And, I said, "Because people like you tell me." My view of the media and the news is quite simple. I learned this from a master teacher. I just need to know enough to know who to pray for.

That is it. So, an easy solution for wellness is turn off the news.

Also, mute or change the channel when the pharmaceutical ads come on. **Pharmaceutical ads are not healthy to your wellness. Every thought is a prayer.** The last thought you want in your mind, consciously or unconsciously, real or unreal, is the idea that there's this pill to fix this thing and even if it fixes the thing, you'll have these side effects, and that gets buried in either the conscious or unconscious state, which means, there a chance that you manifest it? Yes. If you did not know it exists, would you be likely to manifest it? No.

Pharmaceutical ads give you the idea to manifest an issue, and not only manifest the issue, but manifest the pill, and manifest the side effects. Where is the health in that? Where is the wellness in that whole idea? How hard is it for you to either change the channel when it comes on or mute it? Do not expose yourself to those TV ads.

Why do you think the pharmaceutical companies have spent billions of dollars? Because, they get more than billions of dollars in return. Why? Because people have manifested the disease! "Oh yeah, that's me. I must be getting that." The next thing you know, they're going to their doctor and asking for it by name. That's what they want you to do. They understand the process. They know if they advertise it, people will ask for it by name. **People begin to get the symptoms.**

Have you ever thought, with the pharmaceutical companies and all the technology and what they call modern medicine, do we have more disease or less disease? Do we have less disease today that we had in the past? No. So, a very simple solution, is to turn off the news and either change the channel or mute the pharmaceutical ads.

Another idea, **don't allow people around you to talk about medical issues.** What happens is when people are discussing their medical issues, it becomes a focal part of the conversation, becomes the **focal part of their identity**. They're no longer this person. They are now this new person with the "issue" and because of the "issue," they get attention. They have something to talk about. They're somebody now or they think they're somebody now.

The last thing you want entering into your conscious or unconscious idea is an identity with a physical issue. Let's look at our example of when a person yawns and another person on the other side of the room starts yawning. What went across the room? **The idea**. Looking back at our sneeze example, do you think it's any different when somebody coughs or sneezes on the other side of the room and next thing you know, somebody on the other side of the room starts coughing and sneezing?

Were there really these "sneezing molecules," some germs that went across the room that infiltrated a body that couldn't handle it? That their immune system was so weak it could not deal with whatever got across the room? No. What they couldn't handle was the idea. "This person sneezed, so this means I must get this and sneeze."

Well, let's take it up a notch.

This person's yapping about their personal condition, all the treatments they go through and all the "stuff," and all the symptoms and the stuff happening, and things falling off and all kinds of things. Where is that going to end? Is it in your conscious? Yes. Is it in your unconscious? Yes.

How healthy is that? Do not...and I mean it when I say it...**do not allow people to discuss their medical, physical issues around you.** That is not conducive for your wellness. In fact, it's quite the opposite and **you're not helping them**. You are fueling their fire and reinforcing their identity. There's no benefit in it. This why throughout this book the term "issue" is used instead of using a medical term.

Number three, **be the observer of your thoughts,** thoughts are prayers to the Universe.

They're tied to emotions. **Emotions equal your health**. When you become aware of this statement, what exactly do I choose to allow to take away the peace of God of which I can access at any time?

What do I allow to take away my peace?

For wellness, bring awareness to when your peace is jeopardized or compromised, and you minimize it by changing the way in which you respond to it. If less than five times a-year your peace was challenged, it is less likely that dis-ease exist, because you know it, you observe it, you monitor it, and deal with it by changing your view of it to bring you peace.

Not only do you have to observe your thoughts, but you have to observe the spoken words. **Spoken words are commands to the Universe.** The number of times I need to correct clients and patients in the way they are speaking, in the words they choose, because they're literally commanding the opposite of wellness, is often uncountable. Examples are the phrases "that ____ was to die for" or "over my dead body," etc... Be conscious of the words and phrases that are spoken around you and the words and phrases that you use. They are commands to the Universe. The Universe takes it literally and it begins the manifestation process.

Also, the written words, anything you write, **written words are contracts to the Universe** and the Universe takes it literally. So, your bumper stickers, your screen names, things that you write, things that you express in writing are contracts with the Universe, very powerful.

This next key factor for wellness is something that your ego is going to dislike, but if you incorporate this concept, you will be in the state of wellness where dis-ease cannot exist. Using the simple phrase**, "Resist nothing"** brings about a state of wellness. Because, only the things you resist can harm you, and if you don't resist, it cannot cause any harm.

Now, the challenge with this is the ego wants to be in control. The ego has its own plan.

The ego does not like your non-resistance because in its mind, it shows weakness. "Oh, we're not resisting so they must be winning" is what the ego is saying.

Recently, I was completing business transaction, and we were actually foreclosing on a property (we were the lender/mortgage holder), and I was working close with the borrower. We made arrangements for us to gain possession of the property prior to the foreclosure, so we received keys to the property and reinstated the permits. We stabilized the building and made improvements to protect the asset.

It was at this point that I met with the borrower and he said, that he had spoken to his attorney and was told to take back the keys and to take back possession of the property. Now, we just went through this big contractual obligation where we even paid money for these rights! So my response was simply, "Here are the keys."

The borrower then stated that he was going to "go downtown and get the permits to demolish the building." My calm response was, "Fine, knock yourself out. Have fun." His reply was, "And we're going to sue you." I quickly responded with, "You can't sue me because we're not resisting. We're not fighting with you. You want the keys. Here they are. If you want to knock down the building, then knock it down." I then reminded him that the building didn't really belong to me, or to him. Everything belongs to God under the Universal Law of possession. Whatever you want to do is fine. I decided that I wasn't going to give him my peace or buy into the attorney's idea. I later walked away from that table with the keys, with possession of the property, with everything in full force and they did not knock down the building.

So, the idea is if you don't resist it, how can it harm you? It cannot. Resist nothing. You are not in charge. You're just the observer. You're in charge of your thoughts. You're in charge in the way in which you respond to situations, but your ego says, "I can." "I can improve God's plan. I can improve God's creations." Judgment tells you that you can improve individuals, situations, circumstances, and people around you, that you have a better plan than God. The problem is, these ideas do not promote wellness… **they promote dis-ease.**

It's so much easier and so much more peaceful if you resist nothing. You've got to remember that God looks down at everything and sees everything in order. When you look and see everything in order, you too are at peace. When you have that peace, dis-ease cannot occur. Dis-ease cannot even think about being present.

Another factor in dis-ease is **anger.** Anger is your ego trying to control or improve something God created, and this something is **"very good"** as it states in the Bible. And your ego looks at it and says, "No, it's not very good. I know what very good is. Very good would be if they were more like me. Or you and your ego think/say "If I was them, I would be doing it this way," or "How dare they do that?" or "Don't they know who I am?" Anger is your frustration trying to improve God's plan. And you can't improve God's plan.

On the other hand regrets and remorse are the opposite of improving God's plan. Regrets and remorse is your ego saying, "Oh, I did that wrong" which is really saying, "I screwed up God's plan." Here's what you need to understand. Not only is it not your plan, not only is the plan that's in effect greater than anything you can imagine, but best of all is, no matter what you do...

"You cannot screw up God's plan."
It's all in order.

For example, I was dealing with a patient one day who had regrets and remorse issues and he was second-guessing himself on what he did. I responded with this really powerful statement, "You cannot screw up God's plan." Everything is in order. It's your choice on how to view it. It's your choice on how to respond to it.

The fifth idea for wellness comes from a book that I love, *A Course of Miracles*, by The Foundation of Inner Peace and in this wonderful text they have the saying, **"Don't give God's power away."** What is meant by that is, if you don't give anything any power, it can't cause any harm.

With the patients that I work with, I usually break it down this way. "Is there but only one power?" "Yes." "And, is that God's power?" "Yes." Then, depending on their beliefs I ask; "Is that power good?" They say, "Yes." "Is that power love?" Well, if there's only one power, then why do you give God's power away? And, if there's only one power, and that power is good, why do you take that power and give it to something else?"

I see it happening all the time. Right now, one of the biggest segments with the male patients that I work with is that they have a problem with the government. They have problems with Congress. They have a problem with whoever's in office. They have given politicians power. The power of

God. They've taken it from God and given it to something or someone else.

What about cancer? We give it power. The power is based on fear. Somebody tricked you into giving God's power to "it". **Do not give it any of God's Power. It is not your job to give God's Power to anything.** The power of anything other than good, other than love, is **an illusion**. It is something that you have allowed yourself to believe in order to trick you into giving it power, because there's only one power and it's not darkness. Everything ends up going to the light. Everything at some point ends up going back to God.

So, where does darkness come from? We gave it God's power. We did it out of fear. It is really easy to destroy darkness. Bring forth light and you take away darkness's power. It has no power unless you give it power. Light casts out darkness. Darkness cannot exist where there's light. Everything…and I mean it when I say it…everything returns to the light.

For healing, anything that takes peace away, anything that causes concerns, and/or anything that causes fear, take its power away. Even in dealing with my patients and their relationships and family, if they have a spouse or a family member that just "rattles their cage" or takes the peace away out of a patient I'm working with, one of the first things I do is, suggest to the patient to take the power away from that individual and return it to God.

The individuals that you give power to don't deserve the power. You've given that person power, so if they do not have any power, they cannot cause you any harm. For complete wellness wellness, do not give God's power to anyone or anything. It is not your job to give away God's power.

The sixth idea for wellness, is extremely powerful and easy to implement, and that is, when you're the observer, when you're monitoring your peace, when you're waking up and you meditate and you're conscious about the thoughts and the environment around you and the emotions you've tied to each thought, when something challenges you or begins to take your peace away or it takes your peace away, here's what you need to do. **You need to confront all issues immediately at all cost!** The reason why I say immediately is because the longer it goes, the more the issue "festers." The more your body is responding to not being at ease, and the more your body is in this "not at ease" state, the more it increases your chances for dis-ease. So, when I say act on it immediately, I mean act on it immediately. When I say at all cost, I mean at all cost.

I always ask clients and patients "What's your priority?" And they go through their own top three or four, and usually health is in the top three, because if you don't have health, your family doesn't mean anything. If you don't have health, finances don't mean anything. Nothing really means a lot if you do not have health. But what I point out to my patients is that if you do not have any **time**, that's more important than health, because you could have all the health in the world, but if you don't have any time left, health doesn't matter.

Another priority should concern your spiritual being. The spiritual being is the soul essence that occupies the body. If this hadn't been given to you by God, at the beginning of time, you would not exist. The soul is a number one priority, time is number two and then health is number three in priority

If health is truly the number three priority on your chart, then when something comes about, why don't you address it immediately? I hear clients and patients say, "Well, I don't want to hurt the person's feelings. I don't want to confront them. I don't want to avoid them." So, what you're saying is, you'd rather **stuff it in your body and hurt yourself.**

What happens when you stuff it in your body that is tied and buried within you unconsciously and I literally see this in patients. The situation might have happened 70 years ago but the patient is still carrying it. Just by mentioning one word that is tied to the emotion of 70 years ago causes the body to tense up. Their blood pressure increases and the energy in his/her body starts shifting unfavorably. He/she doesn't even know that it is happening.

So, when I say, "Go ahead. Take care of it immediately at all cost," I mean it. There's nothing more important. There's nothing more important that you need to do right this second, and whatever it is, and I don't care what it is, you need to take care of it this moment.

Now, you only have three options in every situation which causes dis-ease, and I learned this from Eckhart Tolle, in his work *The Power of Now*. The 3 options are: 1. You can try to change it 2. You can accept it 3. You can avoid it. If you try to change it, and sometimes you can, you have to learn to put systems in play so it never happens again. You have to be at peace

Second option, **accept that that's the way it is**. Now, there's a book out by Byron Katie, *Loving What Is*, and it breaks down the idea of "accepting" to very simplistic terms. In *Loving What Is*, she says dogs bark, cats meow, guys lay on the couch. It's **what is**. It's the way God created them. It's just what is.

Often, in dealing with patients that have a "problem" with someone else, I show them how the person they're complaining about is no different than…and I would use and animal…and they say, "He just lies around." And I say, "Well, he's like a cat. A cat just lies around." "He never listens to me. "He only sometimes listens to me or conveniently listens to me." And I say, "Still sounds like a cat. A cat lies around. You can tell it something. It may listen to you. It may not. But, if you call it around dinner time, the probability of it getting up and paying attention to you is higher." And, the person says, "Yes, that's my husband." So, I reply, "Well, he's a cat. Are you going to change a cat? No. Are you going to change your husband? No. It's the way God created him."

So, you have a choice to either change or accept the relationship or the person. It's the way God created it. There is nothing wrong with "it" (him, her, an event or object). It's just what is.

If you choose avoidance, you the option to avoid the person, place or thing... at all cost! The reason why is unconsciously or consciously, you don't want to make the decision that you have a fourth choice and that **fourth choice is dis-ease**.

Let me tell you the way it works...

Let's say at work you have a shift in culture. You've got a new CEO, different management style, new boss, new task, whatever, a change of culture, change of something that takes your peace away at work. Your first thing is, "Well, I can't change it. I'm not the CEO. I'm not in charge. So, changing isn't an option." So number two is accepting. "What they're doing isn't right. I can never accept it. It's not right." So, you're left with one last choice and that is to avoid.

Now, to avoid means to go and look for another job. When I'm working with patients that have issues in the work environment (and I have a large percentage of patients that fall into this category) they manifest an illness because they didn't try to change the situation, didn't accept it the way it is, and didn't avoid it. That leaves only on option and that is dis-ease. They no longer have to go to work if they have dis-ease. Disease is a way out. Now, you're probably saying, "Well, are you telling me that people consciously or unconsciously manifest a serious physical condition, so they don't have to go to work?" My answer is yes, this is often the case. I see it every day, and not only do I see it every day, but I see it more than once every day.

I try to assist patients in accepting it, but when we get to that point of, if they can't accept it and if they can't change it because they're not the CEO, or they are not in a position to change it, it leaves them with these options. It's either avoid it, be sick until retirement or no longer be around. I suggest they avoid it. I tell patients, "I would rather you sell coconuts down on the beach, live a simple lifestyle and be at peace." If you don't get up in the morning and you don't look forward to the place you're going, you need to look around.

I recommend to patients to go on the Internet and there's a website called www.InDeed.com, and what you do there at Indeed.com is you type in your zip code and you type in what you're looking for and a gazillion jobs come up. This does two things. It takes the power away from the employer, (fear of loss of job and gives you the option of working elsewhere). How can there be fear of loss of job? There are hundreds of them on the Internet. "I'll just go get another job."

It takes the power away. They've created fear. They've created fear so they could control their employees. Let me tell you that **fear is a fuel for dis-ease.** Now you're going to work being fearful, and if you think about it logistically, the root of all fear is death. For example, some people are afraid of heights because they don't want to fall and die. If the person felt connected to God and felt "One With God" the fear of death would not be present nor would any fear.

The root of all fear is death. So, if you lose your job, you lose your income. If you lose your income, you can't eat, and if you can't eat, you die. So what people do is, as we mentioned, they try to show they have power over you, and this power, this control is evoked by fear, and if they have the fear over you, they can just pull you around like a puppet. The challenge is you won't be at peace, and not at peace is not conducive to wellness.

The workplace is very similar in dealing with relationships. We only have three options. **Change the other person, accept that that's the way they are, or avoid them.** I see patients every day that do not choose those three options, and unconsciously, they jumped up the fourth option. The fourth option is if they manifest a serious condition, often terminal, that they're able to go to a place separate from their spouse and be away and not confront the issue in a hospital, treatment center or death.

The challenge with that in working with those patients is I need to **remove the benefit (yes, benefit)** of having dis-ease. Why would they choose to get better? Why would a patient who is away from their family, spouse, work or whatever situation they do not want to confront or accept, get better? Because they're now at peace, they're away, they avoided. So, what I recommend is to take action immediately. Confront the issues. Face it, take care of it, and remember, you only have three options, because the fourth one is no fun, and if you don't take one of the three options, if you don't try to change it, you don't try to accept it, or you don't try to avoid it, the fourth option is not conducive to wellness.

Now, the number seven key to wellness is the most powerful one, and one that I literally prescribe to almost every client or patient that I work with, and it is the most overlooked. This one technique is worth the price of this book alone, and that is: you need to be at peace right now at all costs. What takes your peace away? Change and accepting it or avoiding it.

But, you also need to see yourself at peace one month from today. More importantly, and this one I use on almost all my clients and patients, and that is, **how do you see yourself one year from today? Are you at peace?** What's around you? And I break it down. What are the family members and how are they? I call it the five F's, family, faith, fun, finances, and fitness. If it's working with a patient, "One year from now, you're totally well, dis-ease free. Yes, you're free of dis-ease. Surrounded by a loving family. You're in a great environment. You love your work, (if you work). You can't wait to get there. You're at ease and you're at peace, and your finances, abundance just flows."

So here's the "Aha"

This is the powerful part. **When you see yourself one year from today at peace (real or unreal),** and **at ease, your body instantly**

responds. Second of all, the **Universe begins to provide everything you need to be in that situation,** and it's an accelerated speed. So, if you see yourself at a beach house, you see yourself selling coconuts, whatever, the opportunities start appearing. The Universe starts getting aligned and whatever you're moving towards starts appearing.

The third thing, and it's the most important thing, and it's my theory, is when you fill your consciousness, remember I said consciousness, with that picture and you hold that in your conscious thought**, the unconscious cannot allow anything in its thought that conflicts with it**. What I mean by that is: if consciously you do not see a picture, you've just given a blank screen to the unconscious to create and do whatever it wants, real or unreal. So, by filling that picture, you're directing the unconscious to go into that direction.

Somebody had asked me, "What are the key things to wellness?" Well there are two things: **meditate, and in meditation, see, live, feel, and experience your life one year from today.**

Chapter Seven Summary
"Seven Ideas For Wellness"

- Meditation
- Avoid News, Medical Ads / Terms
- Observe Your Thoughts
- Resist Nothing
- Don't Give God's Power Away
- Confront Issues Immediately
- Picture Yourself At Peace

** Bonus Class – Learn to meditate online FREE at: http://www.BonusClass.com

Free Meditations (audio Mp3 format):

"Release Negativity" - Now you can release any negativity that you may have attracted.

"Heart Meditation" – Opens closed hearts so that you can give and receive love.

Free at: http://www.BonusClass.com

Chapter Eight

"First Symptom"

In working with patients and clients, I've noticed there's time between first symptom and notifying a doctor of the symptom and that time varies. I'm not telling you not to see a doctor, but I'm telling you, in that time in which you notice or bring awareness or consciousness to the first symptom, real or unreal, when you first get a thought that, "Houston, there may be a problem," at that first thought, here's what I want you to do, and it's very important.

First of all, I want you to **do nothing**. I do not want you to go on the Internet and research anything. I do not want you to think that it's **anything**. I don't want you to tell anyone. I certainly don't want you to label it. I want you to consider it that it is nothing. **If you give it no thought, it's nothing.**

Everything on this planet, or in this Universe or in this realm is nothing until you give it thought. If you give it **no thought, it's nothing**. If it's nothing, it cannot harm you. You don't give it any power. There's only one power and that's God. So, there cannot be any power in this symptom, this condition, or whatever it is that brought it to a conscious awareness.

So, here's what I want you to do. I want you to find somewhere nice and quiet. I want you to set aside a spot, either sitting in a chair or on the floor with a pillow, and I want you to get super quiet and I want you to ask yourself these million-dollar questions: **What exactly is going on in my life right now? What is taking my peace away?**

If you still don't know, reflect on your family, because here is the way it works for wellness. It's either in the family or outside of the family or both. It's that simple. So it is one or the other or both. You need to reflect. If it's outside of the family, is it your workplace? Is it the government? National finances? Things you hear about on the news that you should not be watching? Are you carrying the world?

What are your angers, frustrations, regrets, remorse, chaos, and dislikes that might have recently occurred?

Here's another question. **What change has occurred?** If it's in your workplace, is it a cultural change? You've got a new CEO? Do you have new policies in your workplace? New owner? Did you read or hear about something that's happening nationally or globally that you're not at peace with? Has somebody moved into your house? Has somebody moved out of your house? Are there any issues of betrayal, real or unreal? Is there acting up child or adult? Or, has this child or adult done something to you deep down that you disapprove of? It might be a relationship your child is in, might be your child's career path, and might be something they did that you're not proud of. You need to figure out if there was an event or series of events that you decided on and choose to take your peace away bringing forth the manifestation of the symptom.

If something has not changed, then your "view" of something" (view of a person(s), an event(s) or yourself) has changed.

Once you find this condition, this event, this series of events, whatever it is, you still have only three options, you can **accept it, change it, or avoid it.** Whatever it is it's not more important than your health.

You still do not know…?

If you don't know what is causing the dis-ease, ask God. "God, show me what I need to see." Well, whatever it is, once it's brought to your awareness, **you need to do something about it immediately, right here, right now, at any cost.** Don't let, for example, a family situation shift from peaceful to something negative, which causes the manifestation of dis-ease. Change it, accept it, or avoid it at all cost…just don't let it manifest!

The Benefit of Dis-ease

Unfortunately, and I see this a lot, a benefit of dis-ease is to get another person's attention so they change. You have a choice. Right now, you're at a point where if you get them to change or you can accept them, or you totally avoid them, (either you move or they move), then there is no reason, no benefit for the disease. Because, if somebody moves into your home or somebody moves out, and you are not at peace, (whatever the story is), your body says, or unconsciously says, "This is a benefit. This disease has a benefit."

For wellness you must take the benefit away immediately. Again, you don't tell anybody. You don't look it up on the Internet. This isn't what it's about. You need to **change your view of the situation so you are at peace at all cost.** There is nothing more important. It doesn't matter if you offend someone or if it costs money. It is a cheap investment compared to what you're going to pay physically and financially by not addressing it immediately and allowing it to manifest into an issue. Pay now or pay more later.

I do have patients that have family members or extended family members move into their house. I even had a master teacher, who was thinking of allowing a family member to move in. In that case I said "Don't allow it, do not allow it at any cost." Reach into your pocket and rent them an apartment somewhere else. Do whatever it takes, but you need to obtain peace.

You still do not know what is causing dis-ease?

Now, if you still cannot determine what the issue is, you can do muscle testing, kinesiology, on your own. Just take your index fingers and your thumb, put them together, and then interlock them so they make a chain. So, you've got your thumb and index fingers both connecting and it makes a little chain, a circle, as you pull on it, you ask for a "yes" response and you should not be able to break the chain. Ask for a "no" response and the chain should break. If that works for you, following are a series of questions you can use.

First ask yourself, give me a yes, give me a no, and on the yes, it should be a strong chain, on the no, it should just fall apart. Second question, "Will you tell me about myself? Yes or no?" And, the answer's yes. Next two questions, "Is it inside the family, outside the family, or both? If it's inside the family, is it male or is it female, or both?" And/or "is it me?"

If it's inside the family, you can say, "Is it mother, sister, daughter, aunt," whoever's in your family? "Is it male? Is it about a father, son, uncle, brother, cousin, or nephew?" And, you just go through. If it's outside the family, is it at work? Is it a government, national thing, politicians, workplace, church, club, organization or association? Determine what it is that's taking your peace away.

To begin changing your view of the situation, the first question to ask yourself is, "How does God see it?" **When you see through God's eyes, everything is whole, pure and perfect.** There is no chaos. It's all in order. There's no darkness. **Your manifestation of dis-ease is "in order" you've manifested it** so that you can grow spiritually and deal with a "life lesson". It is perfection that you have this "issue" so that you can learn from it, grow and move forward. God sees everything in order, and is at peace with it. It's God's plan, not yours. So, God looks down and says, "Oh, there's so-and-so, and he's threatened with a medical issue, and how much pain and suffering will the person go through before they change the view of the situation(s) that challenged their peace?"

You need to look and ask yourself, "is it forgiveness? Am I trying to get attention? Am I trying to get priority on another person's chart? Am I trying to gain control over a situation?" These are all benefits of disease. Remember, when you are a child and you have a medical issue, and you stay home from school and you get special treatment, special attention, love, you do not have to go to school, and people listen to every little thing you ask for. You don't forget that, and believe it or not, there's a benefit to disease. You've calculated this benefit, and people actually manifest disease for the benefit. It is done unconsciously, because I doubt they want to do it consciously, but it does appear.

So, you need to turn it around and say, "Well, how does God view this? What's the message? Is it forgiveness? Do I need to surrender? Maybe I don't need to carry the world. It's not my world to carry." And, at all cost, you need to bring it to your awareness. You need to understand that **you are dealing with a life lesson**. You need to get the lesson right away and change the view of it. If it requires action, do it. **Take really big steps to address the situation.** With life lessons, the suffering will repeat and increase until you learn "the lesson." **Learn the lesson right now in this lifetime and end the repeating suffering.**

In meeting with clients and patients, once we have identified what caused it, here's what happens. I ask for the patient to determine if they can accept it, change it, or they can avoid it. And, I don't really care what they choose or what they're comfortable with doing. It doesn't matter to me. If they're going to be at peace, or they believe, real or unreal, that they're going to be at peace, then that's where we need to go. Nothing else and no one else matters. As I have learned from working with Dr. Garcia, "it is all about you."

But, here's the thing...

I ask for the patients **to implement it right then and there.** If they have somebody who moved in with them, and they're not at peace with it, I'll ask them, "Do you have the money to buy them something around the corner or get them an apartment or for you to move somewhere else? And, if you do, do it right now." What patients and clients want to do is they want to put this off. They say, "When I get better, I'll go home and deal with it."

Well, I hate to tell you, what is the benefit of getting better? When they have the disease, they're separated. They're either in the hospital or an alternative clinic, or somewhere else dealing with it. If they pass away, they don't have to deal with it. It's no longer an issue and they don't have to face it. Now, that's a horrible alternative, but it's an alternative that's there, and that's why it has manifested.

So, I mention to every single one of my patients and clients that, "We need to act right away, right now. If you're going to change, if you're going to avoid, or you're going to accept, it needs to begin right now." Because, once you do that, **you begin to heal**. The healing process doesn't kick in until there's peace or future peace or at ease, or a solution or resolution to the event(s) that got them into that condition.

So, here you are with your first symptom.

You're not telling anybody. You're not giving it any power, or labels. It's nothing. Because, if you give it no thought, that's all it is, nothing. You definitely aren't giving it any power because the only power that exists is love, and that's from God. I can assure you that the God you pray to has enough energy, or you can access that energy to be healed of anything at any time instantly and permanently if you turn to the Source, but you first have to identify the event or series of events and change your view of it, or change the condition of it, or totally avoid it at all cost.

Seek the Peace of God

Chapter Eight Summary
"First Symptom"

- **Do Nothing**
- **Give It "No Thought"**
- **Don't Give It Any Power**
- **Get Quiet**
- **Ask - "What Changed?"**
- **Take Immediate Action**

"Still Not Sure?"

Look and see where the issue is on the body.

Back: Finances, money, workplace

Breast: Relationship, family, betrayal, "nesting", attention, importance, appreciation

Brain: Viewed as "not knowing, not intelligent, no longer using "your head"

Throat: Not being heard.

Lung: Smothered by someone, not being heard

Ovarian: Family, "nest", home situation
(Reproductive)

Colon/Bladder: Felt taken advantage of, victim

Stomach: Disliked

Liver: Anger

Prostrate: Fear, victim, mistreatment, "lost ID", finances, "save-the-world"

Pancreas: Recognition, acknowledgement

Skin: Perceived as "ugly"

Note: That it can be a combination of the above such as breast issue that settles in the back could be betrayal at work.

Still Not Sure ... ?
Take the "Self Test" at:
http://www.BonusClass.com

Need More Help?

The College of Spiritual Studies offers Spiritual counseling services, by phone to help you determine the event(s) that may have challenged your Peace and to assist you Spiritually in the prevention or to assist in a Spiritual healing.

Click On "Services" at:
http://www.BonusClass.com
Or call (727) 437-2012

Learn How YOU Can Assist Others
With This Type of Healing
With Our "Facilitator" Course
Visit http://www.BonusClass.com

And click on "Facilitator"

CHAPTER NINE

Why Sharks Do Not Get Cancer

In 1992, William Lane and Linda Comac came out with a book entitled, *"Sharks Don't Get Cancer"* and it tells how it is also believed that the sharks' cartilage can save lives. Well, it is believed that sharks do get cancer, but it's a very, low rate, and my theory is, it's because of the **mindset of a shark**.

First of all, sharks do not have fear. Fear is probably the number one thing that takes people's peace away or they allow it to take their peace away. You cannot have fear and peace together, and sharks don't have fear so it's one less thing they need to worry about.

The other thing is sharks do not know that cancer even exists. Well, if you don't know it exists, you're less likely to manifest it. They do not have it in their thought. Also, sharks do not know and they do not care what their parents died of or passed away from. They do not care what grandparents "got" and what they are going to get through the false beliefs of genetics. That is not in their thought.

Sharks probably do not worry about their diet. They don't worry about exercise. They have no family issues. Family issues are a huge reason why people manifest cancer because they're either mad at their child, their mother, their father, or someone else in the family. While sharks, on the other hand, will eat their young. They don't have family issues. When sharks give birth, the baby sharks are on their own-they are taught nothing.

The number of clients and patients that have an issue of releasing their young is huge. Even when their children are in their twenties, thirties, and up, the parent(s) are not at ease with "releasing their young."

Sharks come together for mating, and then they separate, so there are no betrayal issues. So, there are no issues with children, no issues with parents, no issues with spouses, and all the things that contribute to somebody manifesting or taking away their peace to manifest disease.

Also, there's no news bringing negativity into their thought, so they're basically carefree, and I believe that they must "live in the moment." They're not worried about the past and they're not really concerned about the future. They're just swimming around saying, "In this moment, is there something I need to eat? Something I need to kill? Swim over here. Swim over there. Maybe do this."

My belief is that sharks do not get cancer because they don't have the **"stinking thinking"** we talked about earlier. They didn't allow any other outside influence to mess them up. They don't allow a whole lot of things to take their peace away.

But, the reality is that we are not sharks. We can't eat our young, **but we can choose the way in which we see the world**, and it is a choice. And, when you add spiritual concepts, you can obtain peace.

With Spiritual Concepts, You Can Obtain Peace

Fear is the not knowing what you're connected to. It is the illusion of separation from God. If you really knew that God was by your side, with the power of God, how can anything but good exist? Fear would not be present because it's cast out by Divine love. So, it's a choice. See the God or the good in everything and everyone, and fear cannot exist.

"Hate Nothing"

In dealing with family members, accept that that's the way they are. That's the way God created them. That's the way they're wired. "It's what is." Sure, parents have a role with their children, but what's often forgotten is that the child belongs to God. Under Universal Law of Possession, everything belongs to God. So, when a child challenges you as parent, turn it over to God. When you're challenged by anything, turn it over to God.

When you worry about a child, a family member, a spouse, or another person, it's not seeing that God or the power of God is with that person, and when you see that person connected to the power of God, why would you worry?

When you allow someone to get you mad and upset, it's your ego trying to improve perfection. God made that person that way. God made that situation that way, and you think you can make it better. So, it upsets you. It's your ego trying to improve perfection. God made it this way, so you can't make it better. You think you can make it even better than what God has done.

In addition, you might be comparing yourself with somebody else. "If it was me, I would do this. If I were there, I would have done this. How dare they do it that way?" Well, the good thing is, it's all thoughts, and you can choose which thoughts to have, and when you start deciding the thoughts and you become the gatekeeper of those thoughts and the observer of those thoughts and you cast out fear, you're not upset, you're at peace and you don't allow anything to take your peace away. That's what prevents cancer.

God Bless ...

Mark

Bonus Report

What Can You Do For Others?

- **Bring a new awareness to others seeking healing.**
- **Write a review of this book.**
- **Forward the resources in this book to others.**
- **Bring Peace to anyone with an "issue" to see "it" differently.**
- **Further your education in healing.**
- **Incorporate these findings in the "work" you do with others.**
- **In every situation bring "Light" and "Peace".**
- **Visit: http://www.BonusClass.com**

Additional Resources

Utopia Wellness - 110 State Street, Oldsmar, FL 34677
Phone (727) 799-9060 http://utopiaawaits.com/

College of Spiritual Studies – 18514 US Hwy 19 N, Clearwater, FL 33764 Phone (727) 538-9976
http://www.cms.edu/

For an updated Resource List visit "Resources" at http://www.BonusClass.com

Comment or to reach us by email:
BonusClass@gmail.com

Made in the USA
Charleston, SC
27 March 2013